The Ultimate Keto Vegetarian Book

Healthy and Easy Recipes to Lose Weight and Burn Fat

Lauren Bellisario

Table of Contents

Mexican Tofu Scramble

Preparation time: 34 minutes

Cooking time: 12 minutes

Serving: 4

Nutritional Values (Per Serving):

- Calories: 215
- Total Fat: 16.1 g
- Saturated Fat: 4.5 g
- Total Carbs: 7 g
- Dietary Fiber: 1g
- Sugar:2 g
- Protein:12 g
- Sodium:402 mg

Ingredients:

- 2 tbsp olive oil, for frying
- crumbled 8 oz extra firm tofu, pressed
- 1 green bell pepper, deseeded and finely chopped
- 1 tomato, finely chopped

- 2 tbsp chopped fresh scallions to garnish
- Salt and black pepper to taste
- 1 tsp Mexican-style chili powder
- 3 oz. grated Parmesan cheese

Directions:

1. Heat the olive oil in a medium skillet over medium heat, crumble in the tofu and cook until golden brown, 4 to 6 minutes. Occasionally stir but make sure not to break the tofu into tiny pieces. The goal is to have the tofu looking like scrambled eggs.
2. Stir in the remaining Ingredients and cook until the cheese starts melting, 2 minutes.
3. Dish the food and serve warm.

Classic French Toasts

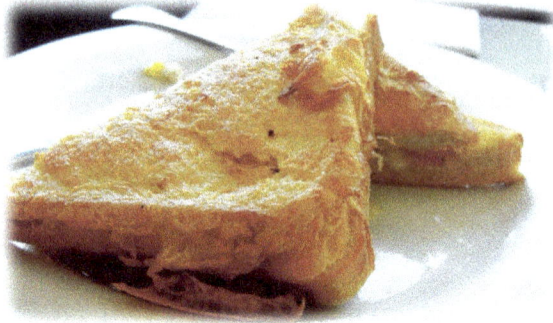

Preparation time: 10 minutes

Cooking time: 6 minutes

Serving: 6 minutes

Nutritional Values (Per Serving):

- Calories: 96
- Total Fat: 9.9g
- Saturated Fat: 6.7g
- Total Carbs: 2g
- Dietary Fiber: 1g
- Sugar: 1g
- Protein: 1g
- Sodium: 66mg

Ingredients:

For the glass dish bread:
- 2 tbsp flax seed meal
- 6 tbsp water
- 1 tsp butter
- 2 tbsp coconut flour
- 2 tbsp almond flour
- 1½ tsp baking powder
- A pinch salt
- 2 tbsp coconut cream

For the toast's batter:
- 2 tbsp flax seed meal
- 6 tbsp water
- 2 tbsp coconut milk
- ½ tsp cinnamon powder + extra for garnishing
- 1 pinch salt
- 2 tbsp butter

Directions:

For the glass dish bread:
1. For the flax egg, whisk both quantities of flax seed powder with mixing water in two separate bowls and leave to soak for 5 minutes.

2. Then, grease a glass dish (for the microwave) with the butter.
3. In another bowl, mix the coconut flour, almond flour, baking powder, and salt.
4. When the flax seed egg is ready, whisk one portion with the coconut cream and add the mixture to the dry Ingredients. Continue whisking until the mixture is smooth with no lumps.
5. Pour the dough into the glass dish and microwave for 2 minutes or until the middle part of the bread is done.
6. Take out and allow the bread to cool. Then, remove the bread and slice in half. Return to the glass dish. For the toast:
7. Whisk the mixture the remaining flax egg with the coconut cream, cinnamon powder, and salt until well combined.
8. Pour the mixture over the bread slices and leave to soak. Turn the bread a few times to soak in as much of the batter.
9. Next, melt the butter in a frying pan and fry the bread slices in the butter on both sides.
10. When golden brown on both sides, transfer the bread to a serving plate, sprinkle with cinnamon powder, and serve immediately with a cup of tea or bulletproof coffee.

Vegan Keto Chao Fan

Preparation time: 10 minutes

Cooking time: 5 minutes

Serves: 4

Nutritional Values (Per Serving):

- Kcal: 234
- Fat: 6 g.
- Protein: 19 g.
- Carbs: 8 g.

Ingredients:

- 1 cup Textured Vegetable Protein, rehydrated
- 300 grams Broccoli, riced in a food processor
- 2 tsp minced Ginger
- 1 Shallot, minced

- 4 cloves Garlic, minced
- ¼ cup Chopped Spring Onions
- 2 tbsp Peanut Oil
- 2 tbsp Tamari

Directions:

1. Heat peanut oil in a wok.
2. Sautee garlic, ginger, and shallots until aromatic.
3. Add hydrated TVP and stir for 2 minutes.
4. Add broccoli and stir for another minute.
5. Drizzle in tamari and stir until thoroughly mixed.
6. Stir in chopped spring onions.
7. Season with salt and pepper as needed.

Keto Taco Skillet

Preparation time: 10 minutes

Cooking time: 5 minutes

Serves: 4

Nutritional Values (Per Serving):

Kcal: 171

Fat: 11 g.

Protein: 10 g.

Carbs: 9 g.

Ingredients:

- 1 cup Textured Vegetable Protein
- 1 packet Taco Seasoning Mix
- 2 Tomatoes, diced
- 1 Bell Pepper, sliced into strips

- 3 cups Baby Spinach
- 2 tbsp Avocado Oil

Directions:

1. Stir together TVP and taco seasoning mix in a bowl. Pour in 2 cups of boiling water and leave for 10 minutes.
2. Heat avocado oil in a skillet.
3. Add seasoned TVP and stir for 2-3 minutes.
4. Stir in baby spinach for another minute or until slightly wilted.
5. Season to taste with salt and pepper as needed.

Homemade Vegan Sausages

Preparation time: 10 minutes

Cooking time: 15 minutes

Serves: 4

Nutritional Values (Per Serving):

Kcal: 287

Fat: 11 g.

Protein: 38 g.

Carbs: 9 g.

Ingredients:

- 1 cup Vital Wheat Gluten
- ¼ cup Walnuts
- ¼ cup Minced Onion
- 1 tbsp Minced Garlic
- 1 tsp Cumin Powder

- 1 tsp Smoked Paprika
- ½ tsp Dried Marjoram
- ¼ tsp Dried Oregano
- ¼ tsp Salt
- ¼ tsp Pepper
- ¼ cup Water
- 2 tbsp Olive Oil

Directions:

1. Heat olive oil in a pan. Sautee onions and garlic until soft.
2. Add onions and garlic together with the rest of the ingredients in a food processor. Pulse into a homogenous texture.
3. Shape the mixture as desired.
4. Wrap each sausage in cling film then with aluminum foil.
5. Steam for 30 minutes.
6. Sausages may be later heated up in a pan, in the oven, or on the grill.

Curried Cauliflower Mash

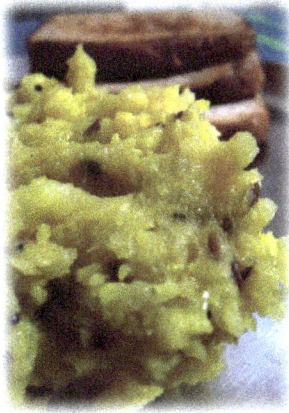

Preparation time: 10 min

Cooking time: 10 min

Serves: 4

Nutritional Values (Per Serving):

- Kcal: 110
- Fat: 8 g.
- Protein: 4 g.
- Carbs: 8 g.

Ingredients:

- 400 grams Cauliflower
- 1 liter Vegetable Stock
- ½ cup Coconut Milk
- 2 tbsp Curry Powder
- 2 tbsp Tamari

Directions:

1. Bring vegetable stock to a boil in a pot.
2. Add cauliflower and simmer until fully tender and all the stock has evaporated.
3. Stir in coconut milk, curry, and tamari.
4. Puree with an immersion blender.
5. Simmer for 1-2 minutes or until slightly thick.
6. Season with salt as needed.

Keto Tofu and Spinach Casserole

Preparation time: 5 min

Cooking time: 5 min

Serves: 4

Nutritional Values (Per Serving):

- Kcal: 222
- Fat: 15 g.
- Protein: 17 g.
- Carbs: 7 g.

Ingredients:

- 1 block Firm Tofu, drained, pressed, and cut into cubes
- 1 Bell Pepper, diced
- ½ White Onion, minced
- 2 tbsp Olive Oil

- 100 grams Fresh Spinach
- ½ cup Diced Tomatoes
- 1 tsp Paprika
- 1 tsp Garlic Powder
- Salt and Pepper to taste

Directions:

1. Combine all ingredients in a pot.
2. Simmer for 5 minutes

Low-Carb Jambalaya

Preparation time: 10 min

Cooking time: 10 min

Serves: 4

- **Nutritional Values (Per Serving):**
- Kcal: 200
- Fat: 15 g.
- Protein: 10 g.
- Carbs: 9 g.

Ingredients:

- 200 grams Seitan Sausages, chopped
- 400 grams Cauliflower, riced
- 1 cup Vegetable Broth
- 1 Red Bell Pepper, diced
- ¼ cup Frozen Peas
- 3 cloves Garlic, minced

- ½ White Onion, diced
- 3 tbsp Olive Oil
- 1 tsp Paprika
- 1 tsp Oregano
- Salt and Pepper, to taste

Directions:

1. Heat olive oil in a pot.
2. Add seitan and sear until slightly brown.
3. Add garlic, onions, and bell pepper. Sautee until aromatic.
4. Add cauliflower, broth, oregano, paprika, salt, and pepper.
5. Simmer for 5 minutes
6. Serve hot.

Chili-Garlic Edamame

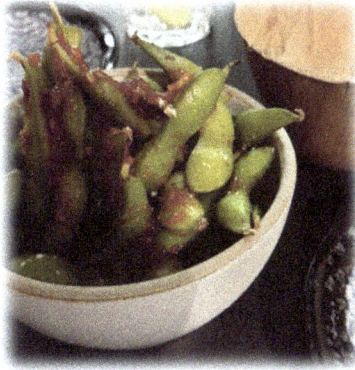

Preparation time: 5 min

Cooking time: 10 min

Serves: 4

Nutritional Values (Per Serving):

- Kcal: 126
- Fat: 7 g.
- Protein: 8 g.
- Carbs: 8 g.

Ingredients:

- 300 grams Edamame Pods
- 1 tbsp Olive Oil
- 3 cloves Garlic, minced
- ½ tsp Red Chili Flakes
- pinch of Salt

Directions:

1. Steam edamame for 5 minutes.
2. Heat olive oil in a pan.
3. Sautee garlic and chili until aromatic.
4. Add in steamed edamame and stir for a minute.
5. Season with salt.

Vegan Potstickers

Preparation time: 25 min

Cooking time: 5 min

Serves: 8

Nutritional Values (Per Serving):

- Kcal: 118
- Fat: 9 g.
- Protein: 9 g.
- Carbs: 5 g.

Ingredients:

- 250 grams Firm Tofu, pressed and crumbled
- ½ cup Diced Shiitake Mushrooms
- ¼ cup Finely Chopped Carrots
- ¼ cup Finely Chopped Spring Onions
- 1 tsp Minced Ginger
- 2 tbsp Soy Sauce

- 1 tbsp Sesame Oil
- 2 tbsp Peanut Oil, plus more for pan-frying
- 1/2 tsp Salt
- ½ tsp Pepper
- 250 grams Green Cabbage

Directions:

1. Heat peanut oil in a pan. Sautee minced ginger and spring onions until aromatic.
2. Add tofu, mushrooms, and carrots. Sautee for 2-3 minutes.
3. Take off the heat and season with soy sauce, sesame oil, salt, and pepper.
4. Blanch cabbage leaves in boiling water to soften.
5. Lay a piece cabbage leaf on your chopping board. Fill with about a tablespoon of the tofu mixture. Fold and secure with toothpicks.
6. Repeat for remaining ingredients.
7. Heat about 2 tbsp of peanut oil in a pan. Arrange dumplings in and fry for 2 minutes over medium heat.
8. Add about a quarter cup of water into the pan and cover. Steam over low heat until all water has evaporated.

Glazed Carrots

Preparation time: 10 minutes

Cooking time: 4 hours

Servings: 10

Nutritional Values (Per Serving):

- Calories 159
- Fat 4
- Fiber 4
- Carbs 30
- Protein 2

Ingredients:

- 1 pound parsnips, cut into medium chunks
- 2 pounds carrots, cut into medium chunks
- 2 tablespoons orange peel, shredded

- 1 cup orange juice
- ½ cup orange marmalade
- ½ cup veggie stock
- 1 tablespoon tapioca, crushed
- A pinch of salt and black pepper
- 3 tablespoons olive oil
- ¼ cup parsley, chopped

Directions:

1. In your slow cooker, mix parsnips with carrots.
2. In a bowl, mix orange peel with orange juice, stock, orange marmalade, tapioca, salt and pepper, whisk and add over carrots.
3. Cover slow cooker and cook everything on High for 4 hours.
4. Add parsley, toss, divide between plates and serve as a side dish.
5. Enjoy!

Mushroom and Peas Risotto

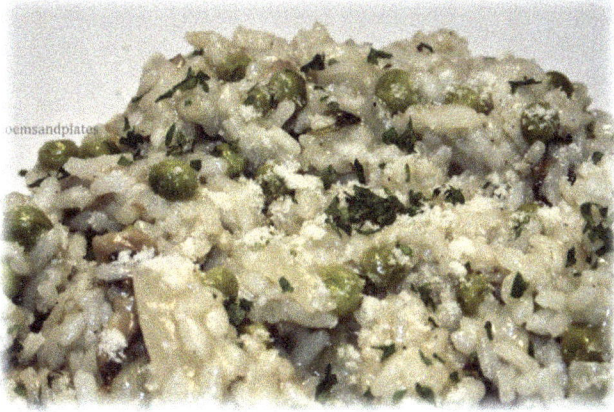

Preparation time: 10 minutes

Cooking time: 1 hour and 30 minutes

Servings: 8

Nutritional Values (Per Serving):

- Calories 254
- Fat 7
- Fiber 3
- Carbs 27
- Protein 7

Ingredients:

- 1 shallot, chopped
- 8 ounces white mushrooms, sliced
- 3 tablespoons olive oil
- 1 teaspoon garlic, minced
- 1 and ¾ cup white rice
- 4 cups veggie stock
- 1 cup peas
- Salt and black pepper to the taste

Directions:

1. In your slow cooker, mix oil with shallot, mushrooms, garlic, rice, stock, peas, salt and pepper, stir, cover and cook on High for 1 hour and 30 minutes.
2. Stir risotto one more time, divide between plates and serve as a side dish.
3. Enjoy!

Squash and Spinach Mix

Preparation time: 10 minutes

Cooking time: 3 hours and 30 minutes

Servings: 12

Nutritional Values (Per Serving):

- Calories 196
- Fat 3
- Fiber 7
- Carbs 36
- Protein 7

Ingredients:

- 10 ounces spinach, torn
- 2 pounds butternut squash, peeled and cubed
- 1 cup barley
- 1 yellow onion, chopped
- 14 ounces veggie stock

- ½ cup water
- A pinch of salt and black pepper to the taste
- 3 garlic cloves, minced

Directions:

1. In your slow cooker, mix squash with spinach, barley, onion, stock, water, salt, pepper and garlic, toss, cover and cook on High for 3 hours and 30 minutes.
2. Divide squash mix on plates and serve as a side dish.
3. Enjoy!

Chickpeas and Veggies

Preparation time: 10 minutes

Cooking time: 8 hours

Servings: 6

Nutritional Values (Per Serving):

- Calories 273
- Fat 7
- Fiber 11
- Carbs 38
- Protein 12

Ingredients:

- 30 ounces canned chickpeas, drained
- 2 tablespoons olive oil
- 2 tablespoons rosemary, chopped
- A pinch of salt and black pepper
- 2 cups cherry tomatoes, halved

- 2 garlic cloves, minced
- 1 cup corn
- 1 pound baby potatoes, peeled and halved
- 12 small baby carrots, peeled
- 28 ounces veggie stock
- 1 yellow onion, cut into medium wedges
- 4 cups baby spinach
- 8 ounces zucchini, sliced

Directions:

1. In your slow cooker, mix chickpeas with oil, rosemary, salt, pepper, cherry tomatoes, garlic, corn, baby potatoes, baby carrots, onion, zucchini, spinach and stock, stir, cover and cook on Low for 8 hours.
2. Divide everything between plates and serve as a side dish.
3. Enjoy!

Eggplant and Kale Mix

Preparation time: 10 minutes

Cooking time: 2 hours

Servings: 6

Nutritional Values (Per Serving):

- Calories 251
- Fat 9
- Fiber 6
- Carbs 34
- Protein 8

Ingredients:

- 14 ounces canned roasted tomatoes and garlic
- 4 cups eggplant, cubed
- 1 yellow bell pepper, chopped
- 1 red onion, cut into medium wedges
- 4 cups kale leaves

- 2 tablespoons olive oil
- 1 teaspoon mustard
- 3 tablespoons red vinegar
- 1 garlic clove, minced
- A pinch of salt and black pepper
- ½ cup basil, chopped

Directions:

1. In your slow cooker, mix eggplant cubes with canned tomatoes, bell pepper and onion, toss, cover and cook on High for 2 hours.
2. Add kale, toss, cover slow cooker and leave aside for now.
3. Meanwhile, in a bowl, mix oil with vinegar, mustard, garlic, salt and pepper and whisk well.
4. Add this over eggplant mix, also add basil, toss, divide between plates and serve as a side dish.
5. Enjoy!

Thai Veggie Mix

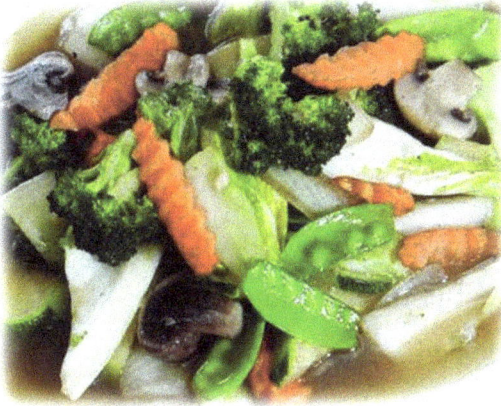

Preparation time: 10 minutes

Cooking time: 3 hours

Servings: 8

Nutritional Values (Per Serving):

- Calories 69
- Fat 2
- Fiber 2
- Carbs 8
- Protein 2

Ingredients:

- 8 ounces yellow summer squash, peeled and roughly chopped
- 12 ounces zucchini, halved and sliced
- 2 cups button mushrooms, quartered
- 1 red sweet potatoes, chopped
- 2 leeks, sliced
- 2 tablespoons veggie stock
- 2 garlic cloves, minced
- 2 tablespoon Thai red curry paste
- 1 tablespoon ginger, grated
- 1/3 cup coconut milk
- ¼ cup basil, chopped

Directions:

1. In your slow cooker, mix zucchini with summer squash, mushrooms, red pepper, leeks, garlic, stock, curry paste, ginger, coconut milk and basil, toss, cover and cook on Low for 3 hours.
2. Stir your Thai mix one more time, divide between plates and serve as a side dish.
3. Enjoy!

Simple Potatoes Side Dish

Preparation time: 10 minutes

Cooking time: 3 hours

Servings: 12

Nutritional Values (Per Serving):

- Calories 102
- Fat 2
- Fiber 2
- Carbs 18
- Protein 2

Ingredients:

- 2 tablespoons olive oil
- 3 pounds new potatoes, halved
- 7 garlic cloves, minced
- 1 tablespoon rosemary, chopped
- A pinch of salt and black pepper

Directions:

1. In your slow cooker, mix oil with potatoes, garlic, rosemary, salt and pepper, toss, cover and cook on High for 3 hours.
2. Divide between plates and serve as a side dish.
3. Enjoy!

Green Vegetable Smoothie

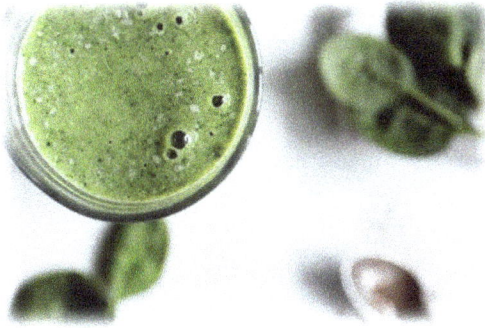

Preparation time: 5 mins

Servings: 4

Nutritional Values (Per Serving):

- Calories: 52
- Fat:2 g
- Carbs:12 g
- Protein:1 g
- Sugars:18 g
- Sodium:36 mg

Ingredients:

- 1 c. cold water
- ½ c. strawberries
- 2 oz. baby spinach 1 lemon juice
- 1 tbsp. fresh mint
- 1 banana
- ½ c. blueberries

Directions:

Put all the ingredients in a juicer or blender and puree.

Garlic Lovers Hummus

Preparation time: 2 mins

Servings: 12

Nutritional Values (Per Serving):

- Calories: 103
- Fat:5 g
- Carbs:11 g
- Protein:4 g
- Sugars:2 g
- Sodium:88 mg

Ingredients:

- 3 tbsps. Freshly squeezed lemon juice
- All-purpose salt-free seasoning
- 3 tbsps. Sesame tahini
- 4 garlic cloves
- 15 oz. no-salt-added garbanzo beans

- 2 tbsps. Olive oil

Directions:

1. Drain garbanzo beans and rinse well.
2. Place all the ingredients in a food processor and pulse until smooth.
3. Serve immediately or cover and refrigerate until serving.

Spinach and Kale Mix

Preparation time: 5 mins

Servings: 4

Nutritional Values (Per Serving):

- Calories: 89
- Fat:3.7 g
- Carbs:12.4 g
- Protein:3.6 g
- Sugars:0 g
- Sodium:50 mg

Ingredients:

- 2 chopped shallots
- 1 c. no-salt-added and chopped canned tomatoes
- 2 c. baby spinach
- 2 minced garlic cloves
- 5 c. torn kale

- 1 tbsp. olive oil

Directions:

1. Heat up a pan with the oil over medium-high heat, add the shallots, stir and sauté for 5 minutes.
2. Add the spinach, kale and the other ingredients, toss, cook for 10 minutes more, divide between plates and serve.

Apples and Cabbage Mix

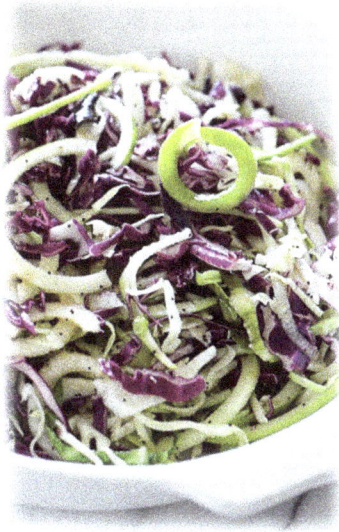

Preparation time: 5 mins

Servings: 4

Nutritional Values (Per Serving):

- Calories: 165
- Fat:7.4 g
- Carbs:26 g
- Protein:2.6 g

- Sugars:2.6 g
- Sodium:19 mg

Ingredients:

- 2 cored and cubed green apples
- 2 tbsps. balsamic vinegar
- ½ tsp. caraway seeds
- 2 tbsps. olive oil
- Black pepper
- 1 shredded red cabbage head

Directions:

1. In a bowl, combine the cabbage with the apples and the other ingredients, toss and serve.

Puréed Broccoli and Cauliflower

Preparation time: 10 minutes

Cooking time: 15 minutes

Servings: 5

Nutritional Values (Per Serving):

- Calories – 230
- Fat – 3
- Fiber – 3
- Carbs – 6
- Protein - 10

Ingredients:

- 1 cauliflower head, separated into florets
- 1 broccoli head, separated into florets
- Salt and ground black pepper, to taste
- 2 garlic cloves, peeled and minced
- 2 bacon slices, chopped

- 2 tablespoons butter

Directions:

2. Heat up a pot with the butter over medium-high heat, add the garlic and bacon, stir, and cook for 3 minutes.
3. Add the cauliflower and broccoli florets, stir, and cook for 2 minutes. Add the water to cover them, cover the pot, and simmer for 10 minutes.
4. Add the salt and pepper, stir again, and blend soup using an immersion blender. Simmer for a couple minutes over medium heat, ladle into bowls, and serve.

Mexican Fideo Soup with Pinto Beans

Preparation time: 5 Minutes

Cooking time: 25 Minutes

Servings: 4

Ingredients:

- 3 tablespoons olive oil
- 1 medium onion, chopped
- 3 garlic cloves, chopped
- 8 ounces fideo, vermicelli, or angel hair pasta, broken into 2-inch pieces
- 1 14.5-ounce can crushed tomatoes
- 1½ cups cooked or 1 15.5-ounce can pinto beans, rinsed and drained
- 1 4-ounce can chopped hot or mild green chiles
- 1 teaspoon ground cumin ½ teaspoon dried oregano

- 6 cups vegetable broth (homemade, store-bought, or water)
- Salt and freshly ground black pepper
- 1/4 cup chopped fresh cilantro, for garnish

Directions:

1. In a large soup pot, heat 1 tablespoon of the oil over medium heat. Add the onion, cover, and cook until soft, about 10 minutes. Stir in the garlic and cook 1 minute longer. Remove the onion mixture with a slotted spoon and set aside.
2. In the same pot, heat the remaining 2 tablespoons of oil over medium heat, add the noodles, and cook until golden, stirring frequently, 5 to 7 minutes. Be careful not to burn the noodles.
3. Stir in the tomatoes, beans, chiles, cumin, oregano, broth, and salt and pepper to taste. Stir in the onion mixture and simmer until the vegetables and noodles are tender, 10 to 15 minutes. Ladle into soup bowls, garnish with cilantro, and serve.

Spinach, Tomato, and Orzo Soup

Preparation time: 10 Minutes

Cooking time: 20 Minutes

Servings: 6

Ingredients:

- 1 tablespoon olive oil
- 1 onion, chopped
- 4 garlic cloves, minced
- 1 (14.5-ounce) can diced Italian tomatoes (preferably with oregano and basil)
- 4 cups low-sodium vegetable broth
- 4 cups water
- 1 teaspoon sea salt
- 1 teaspoon black pepper
- 1 pound uncooked orzo pasta
- 1 (5-ounce) package baby spinach

Directions:

1. Preparing the ingredients
2. Heat the oil in a large stockpot over medium heat. Add the onion and sauté for 3 minutes, or until soft. Add the garlic and sauté for 1 additional minute, or until fragrant. Add the tomatoes with their juice, broth, water, salt, and pepper. Cover the pot and bring to a boil. Reduce the heat to a simmer.
3. Add the orzo and cook, uncovered, for 9 minutes, or until the pasta is tender. Turn off the heat and stir in the spinach until wilted.

Coconut and Curry Soup

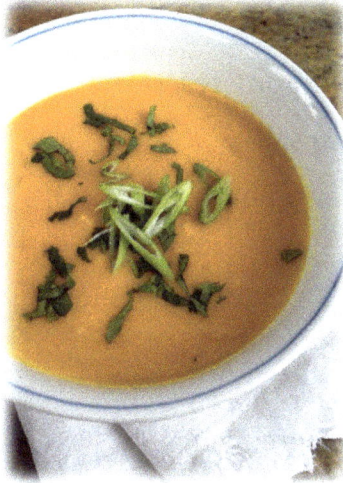

Preparation time: 15 Minutes

Cooking time: 15 Minutes

Servings: 4

Ingredients:

- 1 tablespoon coconut oil
- ½ onion, thinly sliced
- 1 carrot, peeled and julienned
- ½ cup sliced shiitake mushrooms

- 3 garlic cloves, minced
- one 14-ounce can coconut milk
- 1 cup vegetable stock
- juice from 1 lime, or 2 teaspoons lime juice
- ½ teaspoon sea salt
- 2 teaspoons curry powder

Directions:

1. Preparing the ingredients
2. In a large soup pot, heat the coconut oil over medium-high heat until it shimmers. Add the onion, carrot, and mushrooms and cook until soft, about 7 minutes. Stir in the garlic and cook until it is fragrant, about 30 seconds.
3. Add the coconut milk, vegetable stock, lime juice, salt, and curry powder and heat through. Serve immediately.

Creamy Sun-Dried & Parsnip Noodles

Preparation time: 35 minutes

Serving: 4

Nutritional Values (Per Serving):

- Calories:224
- Total Fat: 20.4g
- Saturated Fat:12.2 g
- Total Carbs: 1 g
- Dietary Fiber:0g
- Sugar: 1g
- Protein: 9g
- Sodium:556 mg

Ingredients:

- 3 tbsp butter
- 1 lb tofu, cut into strips
- Salt and black pepper to taste
- 4 large parsnips, peeled and Blade C noodles trimmed
- 1 cup sun dried tomatoes in oil, chopped
- 4 garlic cloves, minced
- 1 ¼ cup coconut cream
- 1 cup shaved parmesan cheese
- ¼ tsp dried basil
- ¼ tsp red chili flakes
- 2 tbsp chopped fresh parsley for garnishing

Directions:

1. Melt 1 tablespoon of butter in a large skillet, season the tofu with salt, black pepper and cook in the butter until brown, and cooked within, 8 to 10 minutes.
2. In another medium skillet, melt the remaining butter and sauté the parsnips until softened, 5 to 7 minutes. Set aside.
3. Stir in the sun-dried tomatoes and garlic into the tofu, cook until fragrant, 1 minute.

4. Reduce the heat to low and stir in the coconut cream and parmesan cheese. Simmer until the cheese melts. Season with the salt, basil, and red chili flakes.
5. Fold in the parsnips until well coated and cook for 2 more minutes.
6. Dish the food into serving plates, garnish with the parsley and serve warm.

Keto Vegan Bacon Carbonara

Preparation time: 30 minutes + overnight chilling time

Serving size: 4

Nutritional Values (Per Serving):

- Calories:456
- Total Fat: 38.2g
- Saturated Fat:14.7g
- Total Carbs:13 g
- Dietary Fiber:3g
- Sugar: 8g
- Protein:16g
- Sodium:604 mg

Ingredients:

For the keto pasta:

- 1 cup shredded mozzarella cheese
- 1 large egg yolk

For the carbonara:

- 4 vegan bacon slices, chopped
- 1¼ cups coconut whipping cream
- ¼ cup mayonnaise
- Salt and black pepper to taste
- 4 egg yolks
- 1 cup grated parmesan cheese + more for garnishing

Directions:

For the pasta:

1. Pour the cheese into a medium safe-microwave bowl and melt in the microwave for 35 minutes or until melted.
2. Take out the bowl and allow cooling for 1 minute only to warm the cheese but not cool completely. Mix in the egg yolk until well combined.
3. Lay a parchment paper on a flat surface, pour the cheese mixture on top and cover with another parchment paper. Using a rolling pin, flatten the dough into 1/8-inch thickness.
4. Take off the parchment paper and cut the dough into thin spaghetti strands. Place in a bowl and refrigerate overnight.

5. When ready to cook, bring 2 cups of water to a boil in medium saucepan and add the pasta.
6. Cook for 40 seconds to 1 minute and then drain through a colander. Run cold water over the pasta and set aside to cool.

For the carbonara:

7. Add the vegan bacon to a medium skillet and cook over medium heat until crispy, 5 minutes. Set aside.
8. Pour the coconut whipping cream into a large pot and allow simmering for 3 to 5 minutes.
9. Whisk in the mayonnaise and season with the salt and black pepper. Cook for 1 minute and spoon 2 tablespoons of the mixture into a medium bowl. Allow cooling and mix in the egg yolks.
10. Pour the mixture into the pot and mix quickly until well combined. Stir in the parmesan cheese to melt and fold in the pasta.
11. Spoon the mixture into serving bowls and garnish with more parmesan cheese. Cook for 1 minute to warm the pasta.
12. Serve immediately.

SALADS

Summer Berries with Fresh Mint

Preparation time: 15 Minutes

Cooking time: 0 Minutes

Servings: 4 To 6

Ingredients:

- 2 tablespoons fresh orange or pineapple juice
- 1 tablespoon fresh lime juice
- 1 tablespoon agave nectar
- 2 teaspoons minced fresh mint
- 2 cups pitted fresh cherries
- 1 cup fresh blueberries
- 1 cup fresh strawberries, hulled and halved
- 1/2 cup fresh blackberries or raspberries

Directions:

1. In a small bowl, combine the orange juice, lime juice, agave nectar, and mint. Set aside.
2. In a large bowl, combine the cherries, blueberries, strawberries, and blackberries. Add the dressing and toss gently to combine. Serve immediately.

Curried Fruit Salad

Preparation time: 15 Minutes

Cooking time: 0 Minutes

Servings: 4 To 6

Ingredients:

- ¾ cup vegan vanilla yogurt
- ¼ cup finely chopped mango chutney
- 1 tablespoon fresh lime juice
- 1 teaspoon mild curry powder
- 1 Fuji or Gala apple, cored and cut into ½-inch dice
- 2 ripe peaches, halved, pitted, and cut into ½-inch dice
- 4 ripe black plums, halved and cut into ¼-inch slices
- 1 ripe mango, peeled, pitted, and cut into ½-inch dice
- 1 cup red seedless grapes, halved
- ¼ cup unsweetened toasted shredded coconut
- ¼ cup toasted slivered almonds

Directions:

1. In a small bowl, combine the yogurt, chutney, lime juice, and curry powder and stir until well blended. Set aside.
2. In a large bowl, combine the apple, peaches, plums, mango, grapes, coconut, and almonds. Add the dressing, toss gently to coat, and serve.

Stuffed Avocado

Preparation time: 10 Minutes

Cooking time: 0 Minutes

Servings: 4

Ingredients:

- 2 avocados, halved and pitted
- 1 (15-ounce) can black beans, rinsed and drained
- 1 cup frozen (and thawed) or fresh corn kernels
- ½ cup seeded and diced tomato
- Juice of ½ lime
- 1 tablespoon maple syrup
- 1 teaspoon olive oil
- 2 pinches sea salt
- 2 pinches black pepper
- 1 tablespoon chopped fresh cilantro

Directions:

1. Scoop some avocado flesh from each half with a spoon, leaving a ¼- to ½-inch wall of avocado in the shell.
2. In a large bowl, mix together the scooped-out avocado, beans, corn, tomato, lime juice, maple syrup, oil, salt, pepper, and cilantro until well incorporated.
3. Spoon the filling into the avocado shells and enjoy.

Cherry shed Coconut Muffins

Preparation time: 15 minutes

Cooking time: 30 minutes

Servings: 12

Nutritional Values (Per Serving):

- Calories: 7
- Fat: 14.82g
- Carbs: 5.79g
- Protein: 2.89g

Ingredients:

- ½ c. coconut oil
- 1 c. coconut sugar
- ½ mashed avocado
- 2 c. coconut flour

- 2 tsps. Baking powder
- ½ tsp. salt
- 1 tsp. almond extract
- 1 c. toasted almonds
- 2 c. chopped cherries

Directions:

1. Preheat oven to 375°F. In a bowl, beat coconut butter and Stevia (or coconut sugar). Add a smashed avocado and mix well.
2. In a separate bowl, combine together dry ingredients and add them to the mixture.
3. Stir in almond extract, almonds and cherries.
4. Pour muffin batter into 12 greased muffin cups.
5. Bake muffins for 30 minutes.
6. Serve warm or cold.

Creamy Blackberry Cinnamon Smoothie

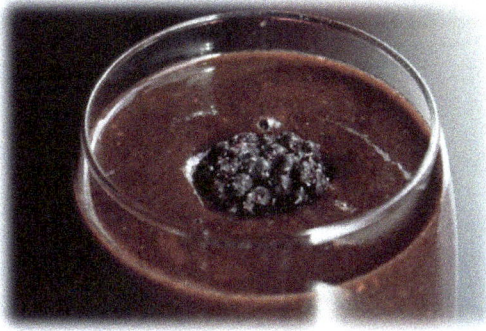

Preparation time: 3 minutes

Cooking time: 0 minutes

Servings: 3

Nutritional Values (Per Serving):

- Calories: 83.78
- Fat: 1.42g
- Carbs: 8.56g
- Protein: 2.97g

Ingredients:

- 1 c. frozen blackberries
- 1 c. unsweetened vanilla almond milk
- ½ c. full fat vanilla yogurt
- 2 tsp. ground cinnamon
- 1 tbsp. arrowroot powder
- 1 tsp. pure vanilla extract
- ½ c. water

Directions:

1. Place all ingredients from the list in your high-speed blender.
2. Blend until smooth and creamy.
3. Decorate with fresh or frozen blackberries and serve.
4. Enjoy!

Dark Coco-Almond Bars

Preparation time: 10 minutes

Cooking time: 0 minutes

Servings: 12

Nutritional Values (Per Serving):

- Calories: 46
- Fat: 30.62g
- Carbs: 7.69g
- Protein: 7.5g

Ingredients:

- 1 c. shredded coconut
- 1 c. almond butter
- 2 c. raw almonds (preferably peeled ones)
- 1 tbsp. coconut flour
- 1 c. melted coconut oil
- 1½ tbsp. Stevia

- 3 oz. dark chocolate
- 1 tbsp. organic vanilla extract
- Salt

Directions:

1. Place almonds in your blender, close the lid, and blend on High for 10 seconds.
2. Pour all of the remaining ingredients, except the chocolate, and pulse until it forms a textured paste.
3. Line a baking sheet with parchment paper.
4. Pour the mixture into pan and lightly press to smooth out.
5. Refrigerate for about 2 hours, until set.
6. Melt the chocolate over a bain-marie (double boiler), and spread it over the bars, smoothing out with spatula until evenly coated.
7. Place back into the refrigerator for about 30 minutes, until the chocolate is set.
8. Cut into 12 bars and serve!

Keto Almond Zucchini Bread

Preparation time: 15 minutes

Cooking time: 35 minutes

Servings: 8

Nutritional Values (Per Serving):

- Calories: 33
- Fat: 7.27g
- Carbs: 8.58g
- Protein: 4.78g

Ingredients:

- 2 eggs
- 1 c. zucchini, grated 1½ c. almond flour
- 1 c. chopped almonds
- ¾ c. Stevia
- 1 tbsp. ground cinnamon
- 1 tsp. pure vanilla extract

- 2 tbsps. coconut oil
- 1 tsp. baking soda Salt

Directions:

1. Preheat oven to 360F degrees.
2. Grease a loaf pan with melted coconut oil and set aside.
3. Whisk the eggs, organic vanilla extract, coconut oil and Stevia in a bowl.
4. With the help of an electric mixer, beat the egg mixture until combined well.
5. Add the almond flour, baking soda, salt and ground cinnamon and continue to mix.
6. Add in grated zucchini and chopped almonds and mix again until all ingredients combined well.
7. Pour the mixture in a prepared loaf pan and bake for 35 minutes.
8. Let cool for 10 minutes, slice and serve.

Light Cabbage Mayo Salad

Preparation time: 5 minutes

Cooking time: 0 minutes

Servings: 2

Nutritional Values (Per Serving):

- Calories: 99.59
- Fat: 3.62g
- Carbs: 6.86g
- Protein: 5.33g

Ingredients:

- ½ medium cabbage head
- Salt
- ¼ c. Mayonnaise gluten-free, grain free
- 2 tbsps. Cheddar cheese

Directions:

1. Wash your cabbage and rinse. The outermost leaves should be removed.
2. Half the cabbage and chop.
3. Place the cabbage in large container and season with salt.
4. Pour mayonnaise and stir well.
5. You can refrigerate salad about one hour before serving.
6. Sprinkle with Cheddar cheese if used and serve.

Peppermint-Cilantro Artichoke Hearts

Preparation time: 10 minutes

Cooking time: 20 minutes

Servings: 4

Nutritional Values (Per Serving):

- Calories: 33
- Fat: 13.77g
- Carbs: 9.47g
- Protein: 5.48

Ingredients:

- 6 artichoke hearts
- 4 minced garlic cloves
- 3 c. water
- 4 tbsps. Extra-virgin olive oil

- 3 tbsps. Chopped peppermint leaves
- 3 tbsps. Chopped cilantro leaves
- 2 tbsps. Lemon juice
- Salt
- Black pepper

Directions:

1. In a deep pan place cleaned artichokes along with water, oil, cilantro leaves, peppermint, lemon juice, and garlic.
2. Season salt and pepper to taste and bring to a boil.
3. Reduce heat and simmer artichokes about 15–20 minutes, turning occasionally.
4. Transfer artichokes to a serving platter and drizzle with some of the cooking liquid.
5. Serve.

Berry and Nuts Dessert

Preparation time: 25 minutes

Ingredients: for 2 portions:

- 10 Oz. yogurt or yogurt drink
- 7 Oz. strawberries, fresh
- Blueberries, raspberries or any berries you may like
- 1 banana, sliced
- Pinch of Pistachio
- Pinch of cashews
- 4 walnuts, shelled
- Pinch of pumpkin seeds
- Pinch of sunflower seeds
- Several fresh mint leaves

Directions:

1. In a serving dish pour the jellied yogurt and top it with all the fresh ingredients.

Pastry with Nuts, Mango and Blueberries

Preparation time: 45 minutes

Ingredients:

For the pastry:

- 1 cup whole wheat flour
- ½ cup whole wheat almond flour
- ½ cup butter
- 2 eggs yolks
- 2 Oz. water
- 12 Oz. blueberries or any berries to your liking
- 2 Mangoes
- 1 pinch of pumpkin seeds
- Sesame and sunflower seeds
- Peanuts, dried

For the filling:

- 8 Oz. cream cheese
- 1 mango, chopped
- ½ icing sugar
- 2 tbsp. lemon juice

Directions:

1. In a bowl mix the flour ingredients with the butter, add the egg yolks and some water until combined and forms a ball.
2. Knead the dough a little until it is smooth and refrigerate for half an hour covered with a napkin.
3. Mix all the ingredients of the pastry filling in a blender.
4. Grease your baking tray or a cooking tin and dust with some flour.
5. Pour the dough into the tin and bake for 30 minutes (200 grades) until lightly brown.
6. Pour the filling onto the pastry and top it with berries and nuts. Add some dessert sauce for serving.

Keto Vegan Pumpkin Mousse

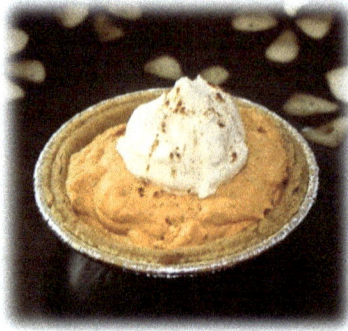

Preparation time: 15 minutes

Ingredients:

- 15 oz. firm Tofu
- 15 oz. organic Pumpkin
- 1 tbsp. Cinnamon
- ½ tsp. Ginger
- Stevia for sweetening

Directions:

1. Mix all the ingredients in a blender until smooth. Taste and add more stevia for sweetening.

Keto Flax Seed Waffles

Preparation time: 20 minutes

Ingredients: for 4 portions:

- 2 cups Golden Flax Seed
- 1 tbsp. Baking Powder
- 5 tbsp. Flax Seed Meal (mixed with 15 tbsp. Water)
- ⅓ cup Avocado Oil
- ½ cup Water
- 1 tsp. Sea Salt
- 1 tbsp. fresh Herbs (thyme, rosemary or parsley) or 2 tsp. cinnamon, ground

Directions:

1. Preheat the waffle-maker.
2. Combine the flax seed with baking powder with a pinch of salt in a bowl. Whisk the mixture.
3. Place the jelly-like flax seed mixture, some water and oil into the blender and pulse until foamy.

4. Transfer the liquid mixture to the bowl with the flax seed mixture. Stir until combined. The mixture must be fluffy.

5. Once it is combined, set aside for a couple of minutes. Add some fresh herbs or cinnamon. Divide the mixture into 4 servings.

6. Scoop each, one at a time, onto the waffle maker. Cook with the closed top until it's ready. Repeat with the remaining batter.

7. Eat immediately or keep in an air-tight container for a couple of weeks.

Keto Lemon Fat Bombs

Preparation time: 60 minutes

Ingredients (for approx. 30 fat bombs):

- 1 cup Coconut Oil, melted
- 2 cups Raw Cashews, boiled for 10 minutes, soaked
- ½ cup Coconut Butter
- 1 Lemon Zest
- 2 Lemons, juiced
- ¼ cup Coconut Flour
- ⅓ cup Coconut, shredded
- A pinch of salt
- Stevia for sweetening

Directions:

1. Mix all the ingredients in a food processor and blend until combined.
2. Place the mixture to a bowl and have it cooled up in the freezer to 40 minutes.

3. Remove from freezer and make the balls.
4. Place them onto the cooking tray and again place into the freezer for hardening.
5. Remove from the freezer and store in an air-tight container for up to a week. Let them thaw before serving.

Candied Pecans

Preparation time: 60 minutes

Ingredients for 4 portions:

- 6 oz. Whole Pecans
- ½ cup Aquafaba
- 1 oz. Palm Sugar
- 1 oz. whole Green Cardamom Pods
- ¼ tsp. Salt
- 1 tsp. Allspice

Directions:

1. Pre-heat oven to 350°F/180°C.
2. Prepare a baking tray with a piece of parchment paper.
3. Remove the cardamom seeds from the pods. Crush the seeds and lay them onto one side of the tray.
4. Chop the sugar or grind it in a food processor.

5. Whisk the aquafaba until frothy, stir in the sugar and salt. Fold in the nuts, allspice, cardamom, until everything is coated.
6. Spread the mixture evenly over the baking tray for about 15 minutes and replace it onto the cooling rack.
7. When cooled, pecans can be enjoyed as a topping or as they are.

Rice and Cantaloupe Ramekins

Preparation time: 10 minutes

Cooking time: 30 minutes

Servings: 4

Nutritional Values (Per Serving):

- Calories 180
- Fat 5.3
- Fiber 5.4
- Carbs 11.5
- Protein 4

Ingredients:

- 2 tablespoons flaxseed mixed with 3 tablespoons water
- 2 cups cauliflower rice, steamed
- 1 cup coconut cream
- 2 tablespoons stevia
- 1 teaspoon vanilla extract

- ½ cup cantaloupe, peeled and chopped
- Cooking spray

Directions:

1. In a bowl, mix the cauliflower rice with the flaxseed mix and the other ingredients except the cooking spray and whisk well.
2. Grease 4 ramekins with the cooking spray, divide the rice mix in each and cook at 360 degrees F for 30 minutes.
3. Serve cold.

Strawberries Cream

Preparation time: 10 minutes

Cooking time: 0 minutes

Servings: 2

Nutritional Values (Per Serving):

- Calories 182
- Fat 3.1
- Fiber 2.3
- Carbs 3.5
- Protein 2

Ingredients:

- 1 cup strawberries, chopped
- 1 cup coconut cream
- 1 tablespoon stevia
- ½ teaspoon vanilla extract

Directions:

1. In a blender, combine the strawberries with the cream and the other ingredients, pulse well, divide into cups and serve cold.

Smokey Cheddar Cheese (vegan)

Preparation time: 20 minutes

Cooking time: 0 minute

Servings: 8

Nutritions:

- Calories: 249 kcal
- Net Carbs: 6.9g
- Fat: 21.7g
- Protein: 6.1g
- Fiber: 4.3g
- Sugar: 2.6g

Ingredients:

- 1 cup raw cashews (unsalted)
- 1 cup macadamia nuts (unsalted)
- 4 tsp. tapioca starch
- 1 cup water
- ¼ cup fresh lime juice
- ¼ cup tahini
- ½ tsp. liquid smoke
- ¼ cup paprika powder
- ½ tsp. ground mustard seeds
- 2 tbsp. onion powder
- 1 tsp. Himalayan salt
- ½ tsp. chili powder
- 1 tbsp. coconut oil

Directions:

1. Cover the cashews with water in a small bowl and let sit for 4 to 6 hours. Rinse and drain the cashews after soaking. Make sure no water is left.
2. Mix the tapioca starch with the cup of water in a small saucepan. Heat the pan over medium heat.

3. Bring the water with tapioca starch to a boil. After 1 minute, take the pan off the heat and set the mixture aside to cool down.
4. Put all the remaining ingredients—except the coconut oil—in a blender or food processor. Blend until these ingredients are combined into a smooth mixture.
5. Stir in the tapioca starch with water and blend again until all ingredients: have fully incorporated.
6. Grease a medium-sized bowl with the coconut oil to prevent the cheese from sticking to the edges. Gently pour the mixture into the bowl.
7. Refrigerate the bowl, uncovered, for about 3 hours until the cheese is firm and ready to enjoy!
8. Alternatively, store the cheese in an airtight container in the fridge and consume within 6 days. Store for a maximum of 60 days in the freezer and thaw at room temperature.

Mozzarella Cheese (vegan)

Preparation time: 20 minutes

Cooking time: 0 minute

Servings: 16

Nutritions:

- Calories: 101kcal
- Net Carbs: 2.1g
- Fat: 9.2g
- Protein: 2.2g
- Fiber: 0.9g
- Sugar: 0.9g

Ingredients:

- 1 cup raw cashews (unsalted)
- ½ cup macadamia nuts (unsalted)
- ½ cup pine nuts
- ½ cup water

- ½ tbsp. coconut oil
- ½ tsp. light miso paste
- 2 tbsp. agar-agar
- 1 tsp. fresh lime juice
- 1 tsp. Himalayan salt

Directions:

1. Cover the cashews with water in a small bowl and let sit for 4 to 6 hours. Rinse and drain the cashews after soaking. Make sure no water is left.
2. Mix the agar-agar with the ½ cup of water in a small saucepan. Put the pan over medium heat.
3. Bring the agar-agar mixture to a boil. After 1 minute, take it off the heat and set the mixture aside to cool down.
4. Put all the other ingredients—except the coconut oil—in a blender or food processor. Blend until everything is well combined.
5. Add the agar-agar with water and blend again until all ingredients have been fully incorporated.
6. Grease a medium-sized bowl with the coconut oil to prevent the cheese from sticking to the edges. Gently transfer the cheese mixture into the bowl by using a spatula.

7. Refrigerate the bowl, uncovered, for about 3 hours until the cheese is firm; then serve and enjoy!
8. Alternatively, store the cheese in an airtight container in the fridge. Consume within 6 days. Store for a maximum of 60 days in the freezer and thaw at room temperature.

Feta Cheese (vegan)

Preparation time: 20 minutes

Cooking time: 0 minute

Servings: 4

Nutritions:

- Calories: 101kcal
- Carbs: 5.2g
- Net Carbs: 3.8g
- Fat: 4.9g
- Protein: 10.3g
- Fiber:1.4g
- Sugar: 0.7g

Ingredients:

- 1 13-oz. block extra firm tofu (drained)
- 3 cups water
- ¼ cup apple cider vinegar
- 2 tbsp. dark miso paste
- 1 tsp. ground black pepper

- 2 garlic cloves
- 1 tbsp. sun dried tomatoes (chopped)
- 2 tsp. Himalayan salt

Directions:

1. Cut the tofu into ½-inch cubes and put them into a medium-sized saucepan with 2 cups of water.
2. Bring the water to a boil over medium-high heat, take the pan off the heat immediately, drain half of the water, and set aside to let it cool down.
3. Pour the vinegar, miso paste, pepper, salt, and the remaining 1 cup of water into a blender or food processor. Blend until everything is well combined.
4. Pour the liquid from the blender into an airtight container. Add the garlic cloves, sundried tomatoes, and the tofu (including the water) to the container.
5. Give the feta cheese a good stir and then store in the fridge or freezer for at least 4 hours before serving.
6. Serve with low-carb crackers, or, enjoy this delicious feta cheese in a healthy salad!
7. Alternatively, store the cheese in an airtight container in the fridge and consume within 6 days. Store for a maximum of 30 days in the freezer and thaw at room temperature.

Nut Free Nacho Dip (vegan)

Preparation time: 15 minutes

Cooking time: 0 minute

Servings: 8

Nutritions:

- Calories: 135kcal
- Net Carbs: 3.5g
- Fat: 12.3g
- Protein: 1.8g
- Fiber: 5.4g
- Sugar: 2.7g

Ingredients:

- 1 large eggplant (peeled and cubed)
- 2 medium Hass avocados (peeled, pitted, and halved)
- ¼ cup MCT oil
- 2 tsp. nutritional yeast

- 1 jalapeno pepper
- 1 red onion (diced)
- 1 garlic clove (halved)
- ¼ cup fresh cilantro (chopped)
- 1 tbsp. paprika powder
- 1 tsp. cumin seeds
- 1 tsp. dried oregano
- ½ tsp. Himalayan salt

Directions:

1. Slice the jalapeno in half lengthwise; remove the seeds, stem, and placenta, and discard.
2. Put the jalapeno and all other ingredients in a food processor or blender.
3. Mix everything into a smooth mixture. Use a spatula to scrape down the sides of the blender to make sure everything gets mixed evenly.
4. Transfer the dip to an airtight container.
5. Serve, share, and enjoy!
6. Alternatively, store the cheese in an airtight container in the fridge and consume within 2 days.

Black Olive & Thyme Cheese Spread (vegan)

Preparation time: 25 minutes

Cooking time: 15 minutes

Servings: 16

Nutritions:

- Calories: 118kcal
- Net Carbs: 0.7g
- Fat: 11.9g
- Protein: 2g
- Fiber: 1.4g
- Sugar: 0.7g

Ingredients:

- 1 cup macadamia nuts (unsalted)
- 1 cup pine nuts
- 1 tsp. thyme (finely chopped)

- 1 tsp. rosemary (finely chopped)
- 2 tsp. nutritional yeast
- 1 tsp. Himalayan salt
- 10 black olives (pitted, finely chopped)

Directions:

1. Preheat the oven to 350°F / 175°C, and line a baking sheet with parchment paper.
2. Put the nuts on a baking sheet, and spread them out so they can roast evenly. Transfer the baking sheet to the oven and roast the nuts for about 8 minutes, until slightly browned.
3. Take the nuts out of the oven and set aside for about 4 minutes, allowing them to cool down.
4. Add all ingredients to a blender and process until everything combines into a smooth mixture. Use a spatula to scrape down the sides of the blender container in between blending to make sure everything gets mixed evenly.
5. Serve, share, and enjoy!
6. Alternatively, store the cheese in an airtight container in the fridge and consume within 6 days. Store for a maximum of 60 days in the freezer and thaw at room temperature.

Truffle Parmesan Cheese (vegan)

Preparation time: 30 minutes

Cooking time: 0 minute

Servings: 8

Nutritions:

- Calories: 202kcal
- Net Carbs: 4.4g
- Fat: 18.7g
- Protein: 4g
- Fiber: 1.8g
- Sugar: 1.8g

Ingredients:

- 1 cup macadamia nuts (unsalted)
- 1 cup raw cashews (unsalted)

- 2 garlic cloves
- ½ tbsp. nutritional yeast
- 2 tbsp. truffle oil
- 1 tsp. agar-agar
- 1 tsp. fresh lime juice
- 1 tsp. dark miso paste

Directions:

1. Cover the cashews with water in a small bowl and let sit for 4 to 6 hours. Rinse and drain the cashews after soaking. Make sure no water is left.
2. Preheat the oven to 350°F / 175°C, and line a baking sheet with parchment paper.
3. Put the macadamia nuts on a baking sheet and spread them out, so they can roast evenly.
4. Transfer the baking sheet to the oven and roast the macadamia nuts for about 8 minutes, until slightly browned.
5. Take the nuts out of the oven and set them aside, allowing them to cool down.
6. Grease a medium-sized shallow baking dish with ½ tablespoon of truffle oil.

7. Add the soaked cashews, roasted macadamia nuts, and all the remaining ingredients to a blender or food processor. Blend everything into a crumbly mixture.
8. Transfer the crumbly parmesan into the baking dish, spread it out evenly, and firmly press it down until it has fused together into an even layer of cheese.
9. Cover the baking dish with aluminum foil and refrigerate the cheese for 8 hours or until the parmesan is firm.
10. Serve or store the cheese in an airtight container in the fridge and consume within 6 days. Store for a maximum of 60 days
11. in the freezer and thaw at room temperature.

www.Ingramcontent.com/pod-product-compliance
Lightning Source LLC
Chambersburg PA
CBHW050756030426
42336CB00012B/1840